Embrace the Change

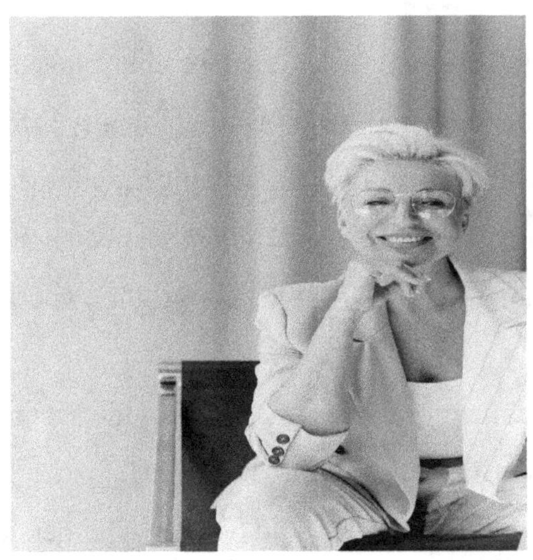

A Woman's Guide to Menopause and Beyond

Mika Wole

Copyright ©2023 Mika Wole

This publication is designed to provide accurate and authoritative information in regard to the subject matter covered. It is sold with the understanding that the publisher is not engaged in rendering legal, accounting, or other professional services. If legal advice or other expert assistance is required, the services of a competent professional should be sought.

INTRODUCTION

Once upon a time, there lived a group of women at various stages of life. Some were mothers, some were grandmothers, and others were simply navigating the twists and turns of womanhood. Despite their diverse paths, they shared a common bond: the journey through menopause.

Among them was Sarah, a vibrant woman in her early fifties, who found herself grappling with the bewildering changes that menopause brought. Sleepless nights, sudden hot flashes, and unpredictable mood swings had become her unwelcome companions. Feeling lost and overwhelmed, Sarah yearned for guidance and understanding.

It was during one of her restless nights that Sarah stumbled upon a book titled "Embrace the

Change: A Woman's Guide to Menopause and Beyond." Intrigued by the promise of support and insight, she eagerly delved into its pages. What she discovered within those chapters was nothing short of transformative.

With each turn of the page, Sarah found herself enveloped in a world of understanding and empathy. The book gently illuminated the complexities of menopause, offering practical advice, soothing words, and a sense of belonging. From nutrition tips to coping strategies for mood swings, Sarah found solace in the wisdom shared within its pages.

Armed with newfound knowledge and empowered by the support of her fellow women, Sarah embarked on a journey of self-discovery and renewal. She embraced the changes of menopause with grace and resilience, knowing that she was not alone in her quest for health and happiness.

As you embark on the pages of this book, may you find comfort, inspiration, and companionship in the stories within. Together, we can navigate the challenges of menopause with grace, dignity, and an unwavering spirit of resilience.

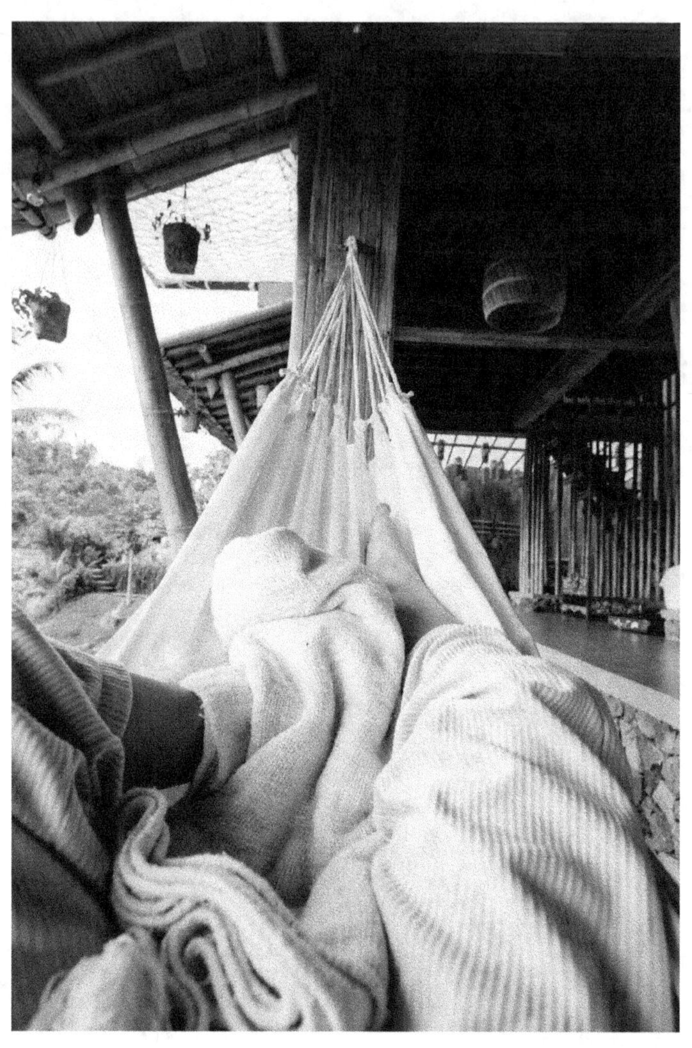

Chapter 1: The Menopausal Transition

What is Menopause?

Menopause is a natural process that marks the end of a woman's reproductive times. It's characterised by the cessation of menstruation and the decline in hormone production, particularly estrogen and progesterone, by the ovaries. While menopause is a normal and ineluctable part of a woman's life cycle, it frequently brings about a range of physical, emotional, and hormonal changes. The trip through menopause generally begins with a phase called perimenopause, which can last for several years before menopause itself occurs. This is characterised by irregular menstrual cycles, fluctuating hormone levels, and the onset of menopausal symptoms similar to hot flashes, night sweats, mood swings, and changes in libido.   Menopause generally occurs between the periods of 45 and 55, with the average age being around 51 in most women. Still, the timing of menopause can vary extensively among individuals, told by factors similar to genetics, life, reproductive history, and overall health. Some women may witness menopause before due to medical conditions, surgical interventions(such as hysterectomy), or certain life factors(such as smoking).

Perimenopause: Understanding the Transition Phase

Perimenopause is like a warm- up before the main event – menopause. It's a time when your body starts to make changes, getting ready for the big shift ahead. Think of it as your body's way of easing into menopause, like dipping your toe in the water before diving in.

During perimenopause, which can last for several years before menopause officially kicks in, your ovaries start to produce less estrogen and your menstrual cycle becomes irregular. occasionally you might have a period one month and then skip the next. Other times, your periods might come heavier or lighter than usual.   You might also start to notice some pesky symptoms like hot flashes, night sweats, mood swings, and trouble sleeping. These symptoms can vary from woman to woman, and they can occasionally catch you off guard. One second you are feeling fine, and the next minute, you are sweating like you've just run a marathon!   But do not worry, you are not alone. numerous women witness these changes during perimenopause, and it's all part of the natural process of getting aged. Your body is just conforming to the new normal, and it might take some time to get used to it.

Understanding perimenopause is the first step in managing its symptoms and navigating this transition phase with ease. By knowing what to anticipate and how to manage with the changes, you can embrace perimenopause as a natural part of life and focus on staying healthy and happy during this time.

Signs and Symptoms of Menopause

1. Hot Flashes and Night Sweats

One of the most common symptoms of menopause is hot flashes. A hot flash is an unforeseen feeling of warmth that spreads over the body, frequently accompanied by flushing of the face and sweating. Night sweats are similar to hot flashes but occur during sleep, leading to night- time discomfort and disrupted sleep patterns.

2. Irregular Periods

As women approach menopause, their menstrual cycles may become irregular. Periods may become shorter or longer in duration, and the flow may become lighter or heavier. Some women may witness skipped periods or spotting between periods.

3. Vaginal Dryness and Discomfort

Decreased estrogen levels during menopause can lead to vaginal dryness, itching, and discomfort. This can result in pain or discomfort during sexual intercourse, affecting sexual health and intimacy.

4. Mood Swings and Emotional Changes

Hormonal fluctuations during menopause can affect mood and emotional well- being. Some women may witness mood swings, irritability, anxiety, or depression. These emotional changes can impact daily life and relationships.

5. Sleep Disturbances

Numerous women experience sleep disturbances during menopause, including insomnia and disrupted sleep patterns. Night sweats and hot flashes can contribute to sleep problems, leading to fatigue and day sleepiness.

6. Changes in Libido

Changes in hormone levels can affect sexual desire and libido during menopause. Some women may witness a decrease in libido, while others may have an increase in sexual desire. Vaginal dryness and discomfort can also affect sexual health and intimacy.

7. Weight Gain

Weight gain is common during menopause, particularly around the tummy. Changes in metabolism and hormonal fluctuations can contribute to weight gain, despite maintaining the same diet and exercise routine.

8. Cognitive Changes

Some women may witness cognitive changes during menopause, similar to difficulty concentrating, memory problems, or brain fog. These changes can be frustrating but are generally temporary.

9. Hair and Skin Changes

Changes in hormone levels during menopause can affect hair and skin health. Some women may witness hair thinning or loss, while others may notice changes in skin texture, such as dryness or acne.

10. Bone Loss and Osteoporosis

Estrogen plays a crucial part in maintaining bone density, so the decline in estrogen levels during menopause can increase the threat of osteoporosis and bone fractures. It's essential to prioritise bone health during menopause through diet, exercise, and supplementation if necessary.

Chapter 2: Hormones and Health

During menopause, women witness significant hormonal changes that can affect their health and well- being. These changes are a natural part of the ageing process and can lead to various symptoms and challenges. Let's explore how hormones change during menopause and their impact on overall health.

Hormonal Changes During Menopause

Menopause is characterised by a decline in estrogen and progesterone levels, which are the primary female sex hormones produced by the ovaries. These hormonal fluctuations can lead to a range of symptoms, including hot flashes, night sweats, vaginal dryness, and mood swings.

Estrogen plays a crucial role in regulating the menstrual cycle, maintaining bone density, and supporting cardiovascular health. As estrogen levels decline during menopause, women may experience changes in their menstrual cycles, ultimately leading to the cessation of period.

Progesterone, another hormone produced by the ovaries, helps regulate the menstrual cycle and prepare the uterus for pregnancy. During menopause, progesterone levels also drop, contributing to irregular periods and other symptoms.

In addition to estrogen and progesterone, other hormones similar to testosterone and follicle-stimulating hormone(FSH) may also change during menopause, leading to changes in libido, mood, and energy levels.

These hormonal changes can have a significant impact on women's health and may contribute to various symptoms and health concerns during menopause. Understanding these changes is essential for effectively managing menopausal symptoms and promoting overall well- being.

Hormone Replacement Therapy: Pros and Cons

Hormone Replacement Therapy(HRT) is a treatment option for managing the symptoms of menopause. It involves taking medication containing hormones, such as estrogen and progesterone, to supplement the body's natural hormone levels. Numerous women consider HRT to alleviate symptoms like hot flashes, night sweats, vaginal dryness, and mood swings. HRT can be a good fit for some women, especially those experiencing severe symptoms that significantly affect their quality of life. It can give relief from menopausal symptoms and improve overall well- being.

Also, HRT may help prevent bone loss and reduce the threat of osteoporosis and fractures associated with declining estrogen situations. Still, HRT also comes with implicit pitfalls and side effects that should be carefully considered. Here are some pros and cons to keep in mind

Pros of Hormone Replacement Therapy

1] Relief from Menopausal Symptoms: HRT can effectively alleviate symptoms like hot flashes, night sweats, and vaginal dryness, improving quality of life for numerous women.

2] Bone Health: Estrogen in HRT can help maintain bone density and reduce the threat of osteoporosis and fractures.

3] Cardiovascular Health: Some studies suggest that HRT may have a defensive effect on the heart and reduce the threat of heart complaints in younger menopausal women.

4] Improved Mood and Well- being: HRT may help stabilise mood swings and ameliorate overall emotional well- being in some women.

Cons of Hormone Replacement Therapy

1] Increased threat of Blood Clots: HRT may slightly increase the threat of blood clots, which can lead to serious conditions like deep vein thrombosis and pulmonary embolism.

2] Bone Cancer Risk: There's evidence suggesting that long- term use of estrogen-progestin combination HRT may slightly increase the threat of bone cancer.

3]Stroke Risk: Some studies have linked HRT, particularly in aged women or those with other risk factors, to a slightly increased risk of stroke.

Other Side Effects of HRT include bloating, breast tenderness, headaches, and nausea in some women.

Before starting HRT, it's essential to discuss the implicit benefits and risks with a healthcare provider. They can help determine if HRT is the right choice for your individual health needs and circumstances. Also, regular follow- up appointments are necessary to monitor for any adverse effects and adjust treatment as needed.

Chapter 3: Nutrition and Menopause

Nutrition and Menopause go hand in hand. What you eat can have a big impact on how you feel during this time of change. Your hormones are shifting, and eating right can help balance them out. This chapter will guide you on how to eat for hormonal balance during menopause.

Eating for Hormonal Balance

When your hormones are going through changes during menopause, it's important to support them with the right kind of food. Eating a balanced diet can help keep your hormones in check and ease some of the symptoms you might be experiencing.

How to Eat

It's not just about eating, but most importantly how you eat. Eating regular meals and snacks throughout the day can help keep your blood sugar levels steady, which can in turn help balance your hormones. Try to include a variety of foods in your diet, focusing on whole grains, lean proteins, healthy fats, and plenty of fruits and vegetables.

What to Eat

Here are some foods that can help support hormonal balance during menopause:

Whole Grains: Foods like brown rice, quinoa, and whole grain breads are rich in fibre and can help regulate blood sugar levels.

Lean Proteins: Include sources like chicken, fish, tofu, and beans in your meals to provide your body with the protein it needs for hormone production and muscle maintenance.

Healthy Fats: Avocados, nuts, seeds, and olive oil are examples of healthy fats that can support hormone production and keep your skin and hair healthy.

Fruits and Vegetables: Be sure to fill half your plate with enough fruits and vegetables at each meal. They're packed with vitamins, minerals, and antioxidants that can help support overall health and hormonal balance.

Omega-3 Fatty Acids: Include fatty fish like salmon, flaxseeds, and walnuts in your diet to get omega-3 fatty acids, which can help reduce inflammation and support hormone balance.

Probiotic Foods: Foods like yoghourt, kefir, and sauerkraut contain beneficial bacteria that can support gut health, which is important for hormone metabolism.

Eating for hormonal balance during menopause doesn't have to be complicated. By focusing on whole, nutrient-dense foods and eating regular meals and snacks, you can support your hormones and feel your best during this transition. Experiment with different foods and listen to your body to find what works best for you.

Nutrient-Rich Foods for Menopause

During menopause, your body may have different nutritional needs. Consuming foods rich in essential nutrients can help address these needs and support your overall health. Let's dive into some nutrient-rich foods that can benefit you during this phase:

1. Calcium-Rich Foods: As estrogen levels decline during menopause, maintaining bone health becomes essential. Calcium-rich foods like dairy products (milk, yoghourt, cheese), leafy greens (kale, spinach, collard greens), and fortified plant-based milk alternatives (soy milk, almond milk) can help support bone strength and reduce the risk of osteoporosis.

2. *Vitamin D Sources:* Vitamin D is crucial for calcium absorption and bone health. While sunlight is a natural source of vitamin D, it may be beneficial to include vitamin D-rich foods in your diet, such as fatty fish (salmon, mackerel, sardines), egg yolks, dairy products, and mushrooms.

3. *Iron-Containing Foods:* Iron is important for maintaining energy levels and preventing anaemia, which can be more common during menopause. Incorporate iron-rich foods like lean meats (chicken, turkey), seafood (oysters, clams), beans and lentils, tofu, spinach, and fortified cereals into your meals.

4. Magnesium-Rich Foods: Magnesium plays a role in muscle function, bone health, and relaxation, making it particularly beneficial during menopause. Include magnesium-rich foods such as nuts and seeds (almonds, pumpkin seeds), leafy greens (spinach, Swiss chard), whole grains (quinoa, brown rice), and legumes (black beans, chickpeas) in your diet.

5. Phytoestrogen Foods: Phytoestrogens are plant compounds that may help alleviate some menopausal symptoms by exerting weak estrogen-like effects in the body. Foods rich in phytoestrogens include soy products (tofu, tempeh, edamame), flaxseeds, sesame seeds, lentils, and whole grains (oats, barley).

6. Antioxidant-Rich Foods: Antioxidants help protect cells from damage caused by free radicals, which may increase during menopause. Include antioxidant-rich foods such as berries (blueberries, strawberries, raspberries), citrus fruits, leafy greens, nuts and seeds, and colourful vegetables (carrots, bell peppers, tomatoes) in your diet to support overall health and reduce inflammation.

Incorporating these nutrient-rich foods into your diet can help support your health and well-being during menopause.Be sure to include variety to each dish, remember, moderation is key! Listen to your body and make adjustments as needed to feel your best during this phase of life.

Meal Planning and Recipes

Meal planning can make eating for hormonal balance during menopause easier and more convenient. By preparing meals ahead of time and having a plan in place, you can ensure that you're getting the nutrients you need to support your hormones. Here are simple meal planning tips and 20 delicious recipes to get you started:

Meal Planning Tips:

Plan Ahead: Take out time every week to plan your meals and snacks. This helps you make healthier and generally better choices and avoid last-minute decisions that may not be as nutritious.

Include variety to your meals: Aim to include a variety of foods from all food classes to your meals. This ensures that you're getting a wide range of nutrients to support your hormonal balance.

Prep Ingredients in Advance: Chop vegetables, cook grains, and prepare proteins ahead of time to make meal assembly quick and easy during the week.

Batch Cook: Consider batch cooking large quantities of meals that you can portion out and freeze for later use. This helps you save time and energy on busy days.

Listen to Your Body: Pay attention to how different foods make you feel and adjust your meal plan accordingly. Your body knows best what it needs to thrive.

20 Delicious Recipes:

Quinoa Breakfast Bowl: Cook quinoa according to package instructions and top with Greek yoghurt, fresh berries, and a drizzle of honey.

Spinach and Feta Omelette: Whisk together eggs and pour into a hot skillet. Add spinach and feta cheese, then fold over and cook until set.

Chicken and Vegetable Stir-Fry: Stir-fry chicken breast strips with bell peppers, broccoli, and snap peas in a sesame soy sauce. Serve over brown rice.

Salmon Salad: Grill or bake salmon fillets and serve over mixed greens with cucumber, cherry tomatoes, and avocado slices.

Mediterranean Quinoa Salad: Toss cooked quinoa with chopped cucumber, cherry tomatoes, Kalamata olives, feta cheese, and a lemon vinaigrette.

Turkey and Veggie Skewers: Thread turkey breast cubes onto skewers with cherry tomatoes, bell peppers, and onions. Grill until cooked through.

Sweet Potato and Black Bean Tacos: Roast sweet potato cubes and serve in corn tortillas with black beans, avocado slices, and salsa.

Lentil Vegetable Soup: Simmer lentils with diced tomatoes, carrots, celery, and spinach in vegetable broth for a comforting soup.

Baked Cod with Asparagus: Season cod fillets with lemon juice, garlic, and herbs, then bake alongside asparagus spears until tender.

Quinoa Stuffed Bell Peppers: Fill halved bell peppers with cooked quinoa, black beans, corn, diced tomatoes, and shredded cheese. Bake until peppers are tender.

Greek Chicken Salad: Toss grilled chicken strips with mixed greens, cucumber, cherry tomatoes, feta cheese, and a Greek yogurt dressing.

Vegetable and Chickpea Curry: Simmer chickpeas with coconut milk, curry paste, and mixed vegetables for a flavorful curry dish. Serve over rice.

Zucchini Noodles with Pesto: Spiralize zucchini into noodles and toss with homemade pesto sauce made from basil, pine nuts, garlic, and olive oil.

Tuna Salad Lettuce Wraps: Mix canned tuna with Greek yoghurt, diced celery, and lemon juice. Take a tablespoon of it into the lettuce leaves and roll up.

Vegetable Frittata: Whisk together eggs with sautéed vegetables like bell peppers, onions, spinach, and mushrooms. Bake until set.

Quinoa and Black Bean Bowl: Combine cooked quinoa with black beans, corn, diced avocado, salsa, and a squeeze of lime juice.

Roasted Vegetable Medley: Toss chopped vegetables like carrots, Brussels sprouts, and cauliflower with olive oil, garlic, and herbs. Roast until tender.

Turkey and Vegetable Chilli: Brown ground turkey with onions, bell peppers, and garlic. Add diced tomatoes, black beans, chili powder, and cumin. Simmer until flavors meld.

Stuffed Portobello Mushrooms: Fill portobello mushroom caps with a mixture of cooked quinoa, spinach, sun-dried tomatoes, and goat cheese. Bake until mushrooms are tender.

Smoothie Berry Bowl: Blend different kinds of frozen berries with Greek yoghourt and almond milk. Pour into a bowl and top with granola, sliced bananas, and chia seeds.

These recipes provide a variety of nutritious and delicious options to support hormonal balance during menopause. Experiment with different flavours and ingredients to find what works best for you and enjoy nourishing your body during this transitional phase.

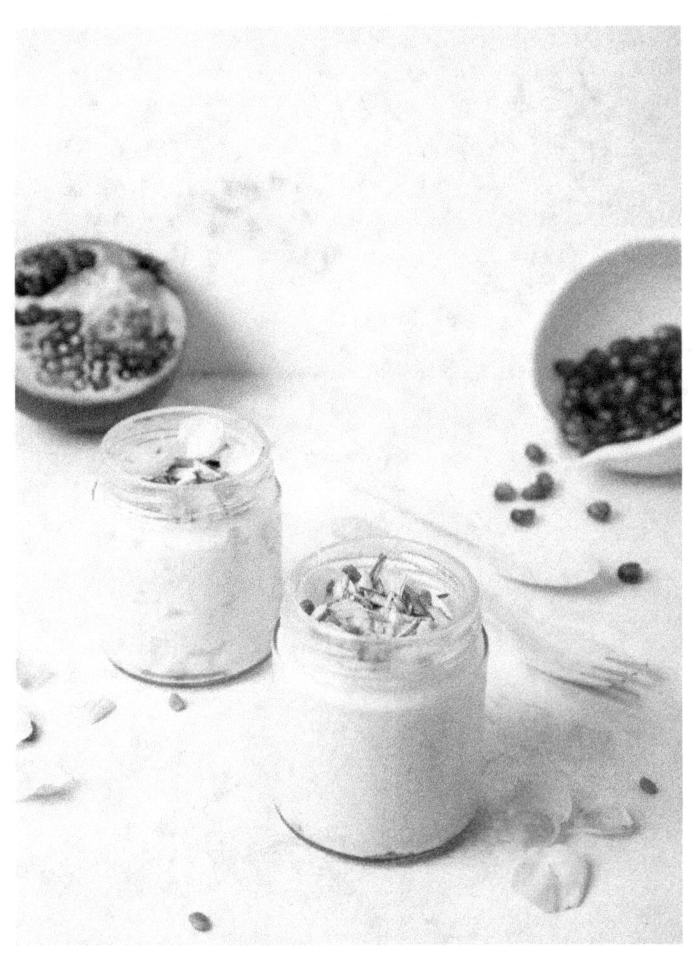

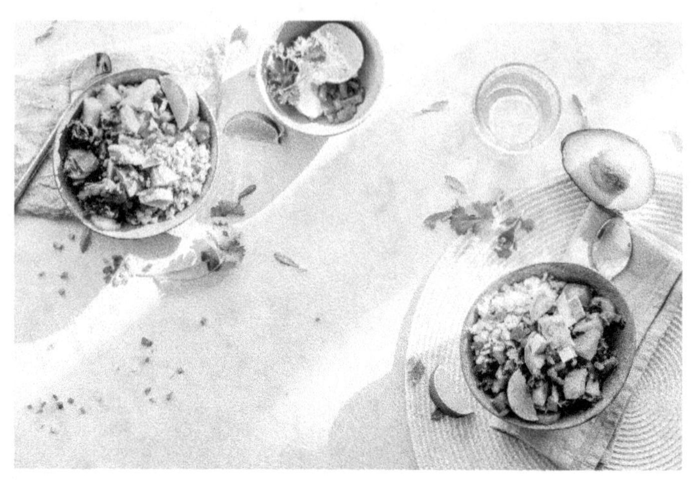

Chapter 4: Managing Weight Gain

Understanding Weight Gain During Menopause

Weight gain during menopause is a common concern among many women. You might have noticed some changes in your body, like your jeans feeling a bit tighter or your favourite shirt not fitting quite the same way. Don't worry, you're not alone, and there's a reason behind it!

Why Women Gain Weight:

During menopause, your body goes through some big changes, especially when it comes to hormones. One of the main hormones involved is estrogen. As your estrogen levels drop, your body might start to store more fat, especially around your belly. This can lead to weight gain, even if you're eating the same way you always have.

The Science Behind It:

It all comes down to your metabolism – that's the way your body turns food into energy. As you get older and your estrogen levels decline, your metabolism can slow down. This means your body might not burn calories as quickly as it used to, making it easier to gain weight.

How Most Women React:

When women notice they're gaining weight during menopause, it can be frustrating and even upsetting. You might feel like your body is betraying you or that you're losing control. Some women might try extreme diets or exercise routines to try to lose the weight quickly. But these drastic measures often aren't sustainable and can even be harmful to your health.

How You Should React:

Instead of feeling discouraged or trying to fight against your body, try to approach weight gain during menopause with understanding and compassion. Remember, it's a natural part of the process, and you're not alone. Focus on making small, sustainable changes to your diet and exercise routine. Try to eat more fruits, vegetables, and whole grains, and find ways to stay active that you enjoy. And most importantly, be kind to yourself – your worth isn't determined by the number on the scale.

By understanding why weight gain happens during menopause and taking a gentle approach to managing it, you can navigate this transition with grace and confidence.

Strategies for Maintaining a Healthy Weight

Maintaining a healthy weight during menopause is important for your overall well-being. Here are some simple strategies to help you manage your weight:

Eat a balanced diet: Fill your plate with a variety of nutrient-rich foods such as fruits, vegetables, whole grains, lean proteins, and healthy fats. Aim for smaller portions and limit your intake of sugary snacks, processed foods, and high-fat meals.

Stay active: Incorporate regular exercise into your daily routine. Choose activities you enjoy, such as walking, swimming, dancing, or yoga.

Aim for at least 30 minutes of moderate-intensity exercise most days of the week to help burn calories and maintain muscle mass.

Stay hydrated: Do this by drinking just enough water throughout the day. Water helps keep you feeling full and may help reduce your appetite. Limit your intake of sugary beverages like soda and juice, which can contribute to weight gain.

Practise mindful eating: Pay attention to your body's hunger and fullness cues. Eat slowly and gently, and stop eating when you feel satisfied, rather than stuffed. Avoid eating in front of any device, it may be a TV or your phone, as this can lead to mindless overeating.

By following these simple strategies, you can help maintain a healthy weight during menopause and support your overall health and well-being. Remember to be patient with yourself and focus on making small, sustainable changes to your lifestyle.

Exercise Routines

Exercise plays a crucial role in maintaining a healthy weight and overall well-being during this phase of life. Let's explore 20 exercise routines that you can incorporate into your daily routine:

Walking: A simple yet effective exercise, walking helps burn calories, improves cardiovascular health, and strengthens bones

Jogging or Running: If you're up for it, jogging or running can be great for burning calories and boosting your mood. Start with shorter intervals and gradually increase your pace and distance.

Cycling: Whether outdoors or on a stationary bike, cycling is a low-impact exercise that improves heart health and leg strength. Try cycling for 30 minutes a few times a week.

Swimming: Swimming is gentle on the joints and offers a full-body workout. Aim for a swim session of 20-30 minutes a few times a week.

Dancing: Dancing is a fun way to burn calories, improve flexibility, and lift your spirits.

Yoga: Yoga helps improve flexibility, balance, and strength while also promoting relaxation and stress relief. Practice yoga poses like downward dog, warrior, and tree pose regularly.

Pilates: Pilates is an exercise that focuses on your core strength, stability, and flexibility.

Incorporate Pilates exercises like the hundred, roll-up, and leg circles into your routine.

Strength Training: Lift weights or use resistance bands to build muscle mass, which can boost metabolism and help with weight management. Target major muscle groups with exercises like squats, lunges, and push-ups.

Interval Training: Juggle high-intensity exercise with periods of rest or lower intensity. This can be done with activities like jumping jacks, burpees, or cycling sprints.

Hiking: Take advantage of the great outdoors and go for a hike. Hiking engages different muscle groups, burns calories, and offers mental health benefits.

Tai Chi: Tai Chi is a gentle martial art that promotes relaxation, balance, and mindfulness.

Practice flowing movements like the cloud hands and brush knee regularly.

Rowing: Whether on a rowing machine or out on the water, rowing provides a full-body workout that improves cardiovascular health and strength.

Kickboxing: Punch and kick your way to fitness with kickboxing workouts. These high-intensity sessions help burn calories and release stress.

Jump Rope: Jumping rope is a simple yet effective cardio exercise that can be done almost anywhere. Start with short intervals and gradually increase your duration.

Stair Climbing: Use stairs at home or find a staircase outdoors for a challenging workout.

Climbing stairs strengthens the lower body and gets your heart rate up.

Barre Workouts: Barre workouts combine elements of ballet, Pilates, and yoga to sculpt and tone muscles. Incorporate exercises like pliés, leg lifts, and arm pulses into your routine.

Group Fitness Classes: Join a group fitness class like Zumba, spinning, or aerobics for motivation and camaraderie while getting a great workout.

Circuit Training: Create a circuit of different exercises targeting various muscle groups. Move through each exercise with minimal rest for a full-body workout.

Resistance Band Exercises: Use resistance bands to add variety to your strength training routine. Perform exercises like bicep curls, lateral raises, and rows with resistance bands.

Balance Exercises: Incorporate balance exercises like single-leg stands, heel-to-toe walks, and yoga balance poses to improve stability.

Remember to listen to your body and choose exercises that you enjoy and feel comfortable with. Start slowly and gradually increase the intensity and duration of your workouts. Consistency is key, so aim to make exercise a regular part of your routine for optimal health and well-being during menopause,

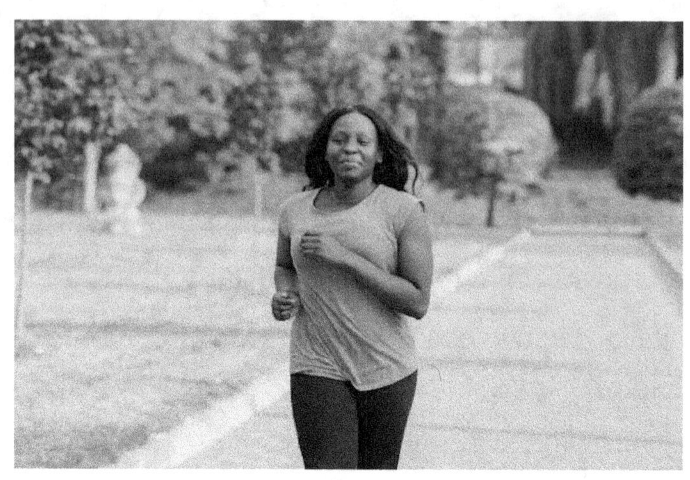

Chapter 5: Coping with Mood Swings and Emotional Changes

In this chapter, we will explore the rollercoaster of emotions that can come with menopause. Understanding mood swings and emotional changes is crucial because they can affect your relationships, work, and overall well-being. Let's delve into why these changes happen and how you can cope with them.

Understanding Mood Swings and Emotional Challenges

Mood swings during menopause are like unexpected guests at a party. One moment you may feel on top of the world, and the next, you're feeling down in the dumps. These swings happen because of hormonal changes in your body. Estrogen and progesterone, two key hormones, take a nosedive during menopause. When these hormones fluctuate, they can mess with your brain chemicals, leading to mood swings.

Understanding mood swings is like having a secret weapon in your arsenal. When you know why you're feeling the way you are, you can better manage your emotions. It's like being the captain of your ship rather than letting the waves toss you around. Plus, when you understand what's going on, you can communicate better with your loved ones. Instead of snapping at them for no reason, you can explain, "Hey, I'm feeling a bit off today because of menopause."

Menopause isn't just about hot flashes and night sweats; it's also an emotional rollercoaster. You may find yourself crying at commercials one moment and laughing hysterically at a bad joke the next. These emotional changes are normal, but they can be challenging to deal with. You might feel like you're losing control of your emotions, but remember, you're not alone. Many women experience these ups and downs during menopause.

Coping Mechanisms and Stress Management Techniques

We're delving into coping mechanisms and stress management techniques to help you navigate mood swings and emotional changes during menopause. Let me introduce you to Grace, a woman who found these techniques invaluable during her menopausal journey.

Grace, like many women, found herself struggling with mood swings and emotional ups and downs as she entered menopause. She felt overwhelmed and frustrated by the sudden changes happening in her body and emotions. However, through trial and error, Grace discovered coping mechanisms and stress management techniques that made a significant difference in how she felt.

Here are 10 coping mechanisms Grace found helpful, along with stories from other women who have used these techniques:

Deep Breathing: Taking slow, deep breaths is a sure way to help calm the mind and reduce stress. Lisa, a friend of Grace,noted that by practicing deep breathing exercises whenever she felt overwhelmed helped her regain control of her emotions.

Journaling: Writing down her thoughts and feelings in a journal helped Grace process her emotions and gain perspective on her menopausal journey. She found that expressing herself through writing provided a sense of relief and clarity.

Physical Activity: Engaging in regular exercise, such as walking, yoga, or dancing, helped her manage her mood swings and boost her overall well-being. She found that physical activity helped release tension and improve her mood.

Seeking Support: Talking to friends, family, or a therapist about her experiences with menopause helped Grace feel less alone and more understood. Knowing that others were going through similar challenges made her feel supported and validated.

Mindfulness Meditation: Practicing mindfulness meditation also helped Lisa become more present in the moment and less reactive to her emotions. She found that taking a few minutes each day to meditate helped her stay calm and centred.

Setting Boundaries: Learning to say no and prioritise your own needs. This helped these women manage their stress levels during menopause. They realised that it was important to take care of themselves.

Creative Outlets: Engaging in creative activities, such as painting, gardening, or crafting, provided a therapeutic outlet for Grace to express herself and relieve stress. She found that immersing herself in creative projects helped distract her from negative thoughts and emotions.

Healthy Lifestyle Choices: Making healthy lifestyle choices, such as eating a balanced diet, getting enough sleep, and avoiding excessive alcohol and caffeine.

Laughter Therapy: Finding humour in everyday situations and sharing laughter with friends helps lighten your mood and reduce stress. It is said that laughter truly is the best medicine during challenging times.

Positive Affirmations: Repeating positive affirmations, such as "I am strong and resilient" or "I embrace change with grace," helped Lisa and Grace cultivate a positive mindset and counter negative self-talk. They found out that affirmations helped boost her confidence and resilience.

In addition to coping mechanisms, here are five stress management techniques to help you navigate the ups and downs of menopause:

Progressive Muscle Relaxation: Tensing and relaxing different muscle groups in your body can help release physical tension and promote relaxation.

Visualisation: Imagining yourself in a peaceful, serene setting can help calm your mind and reduce stress levels.

Time Management: Prioritising tasks and breaking them down into manageable chunks can help prevent feelings of overwhelm and reduce stress.

Self-care Practices: Engaging in activities that nurture your body, mind, and soul, such as taking a bubble bath, reading a book, or practising aromatherapy, can help reduce stress and promote well-being.

Limiting Exposure to Stressors: Identifying sources of stress in your life and taking steps to minimise or avoid them whenever possible can help protect your emotional and mental health.

By incorporating these coping mechanisms and stress management techniques into your daily routine, you can better navigate mood swings and emotional changes during menopause and embrace this transformative phase of life with grace and resilience. Remember, it's okay to seek support from others and prioritise your own well-being during this time. You are not alone in your menopausal journey.

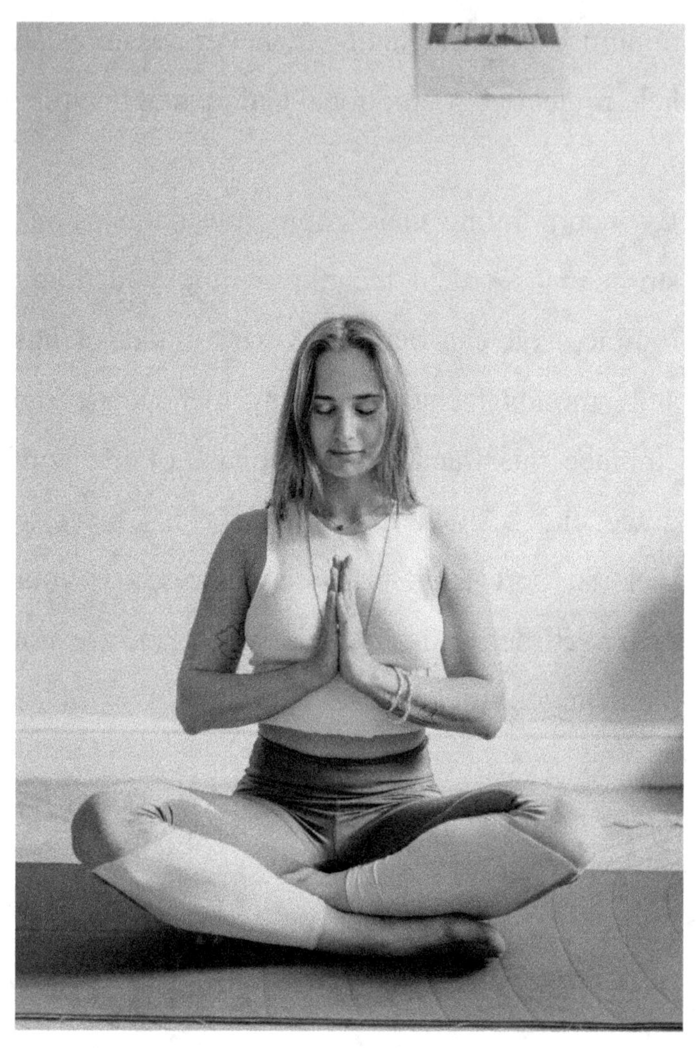

Chapter 6: Enhancing Sleep and Energy

In this chapter, we'll explore strategies to enhance sleep quality and boost energy levels naturally during menopause. Sleep disturbances and fatigue are common challenges during this phase of life, but with the right techniques, you can improve your sleep hygiene and increase your energy levels for a better quality of life.

1. Sleep Hygiene Tips for Menopause

Good sleep hygiene is essential for promoting restful sleep and overall well-being. Here are some tips to improve your sleep hygiene during menopause:

Stick to a regular sleep schedule: Go to bed and wake up at the same time every day, even on weekends, to regulate your body's internal clock.

Create a relaxing bedtime routine: Establish calming activities before bedtime, such as reading, taking a warm bath, or practicing relaxation techniques like deep breathing or meditation.

Make your bedroom conducive to sleep: Keep your bedroom dark, quiet, and cool, and invest in a comfortable mattress and pillows to promote restful sleep.

Limit screen time before bed: Avoid using electronic devices such as smartphones, tablets, or computers before bedtime, as the blue light emitted from screens can disrupt your sleep-wake cycle.

Avoid stimulating substances: Limit caffeine and alcohol intake, especially in the hours leading up to bedtime, as they can interfere with your ability to fall asleep and stay asleep.

2. Managing Insomnia and Sleep Disturbances

Insomnia and other sleep disturbances can be challenging during menopause, but there are strategies to help manage these issues:

Practice relaxation techniques: Engage in relaxation exercises such as progressive muscle relaxation, guided imagery, or mindfulness meditation to promote relaxation and improve sleep quality.

Address underlying health issues: If you're experiencing persistent insomnia or sleep disturbances, consult with your healthcare provider to rule out any underlying medical conditions and explore treatment options.

Consider cognitive-behavioural therapy for insomnia (CBT-I): CBT-I is a highly effective treatment for insomnia that focuses on changing negative thought patterns and behaviours that contribute to sleep difficulties.

Explore natural sleep aids: Certain herbs and supplements, such as valerian root, melatonin, or magnesium, may help promote relaxation and improve sleep quality. However, it's essential to consult with a healthcare professional before using any supplements, especially if you're taking medications or have underlying health conditions.

3. Boosting Energy Levels Naturally

Low energy levels are a common complaint during menopause, but there are natural ways to increase your energy and vitality:

Stay physically active: Regular exercise can boost energy levels, improve sleep quality, and reduce symptoms of fatigue. Aim for at least 30 minutes of moderate-intensity exercise most days of the week, such as walking, cycling, swimming, or yoga.

Eat a balanced diet: Fuel your body with nutritious foods that provide sustained energy throughout the day, such as fruits, vegetables, whole grains, lean proteins, and healthy fats. Avoid snacks that contain a lot of sugar and stay away from refined carbohydrates, which can cause energy crashes.

Stay hydrated: Dehydration can contribute to feelings of fatigue, so be sure to drink plenty of water throughout the day. Limit caffeine and sugary drinks, as they can lead to dehydration and energy fluctuations.

Get sunlight exposure: Spend time outdoors in natural sunlight, especially in the morning, to regulate your body's internal clock and boost energy levels. Sunlight exposure also stimulates the production of vitamin D, which is essential for overall health and vitality.

By incorporating these sleep hygiene tips, managing insomnia and sleep disturbances, and boosting your energy levels naturally, you can improve your quality of life and embrace the changes of menopause with greater ease and vitality.

Chapter 7: Maintaining Sexual Health

In this chapter, we will explore the changes that occur in sexual health during menopause and discuss practical strategies for addressing common issues such as vaginal dryness and discomfort. Additionally, we'll provide five simple strategies for enhancing intimacy and pleasure, helping you maintain a fulfilling and satisfying sex life during this transitional phase.

Changes in Sexual Health During Menopause

During menopause, many women experience changes in their sexual health due to hormonal fluctuations. Decreased estrogen levels can lead to vaginal dryness, thinning of the vaginal tissues, and reduced lubrication, making intercourse uncomfortable or painful. Additionally, changes in hormone levels may affect libido, arousal, and orgasmic response.

Addressing Vaginal Dryness and Discomfort

Vaginal dryness and discomfort are common challenges faced by women during menopause, but there are several strategies to alleviate these symptoms and improve sexual comfort.

One approach is to use over-the-counter or prescription vaginal lubricants and moisturisers to enhance lubrication and reduce friction during intercourse. These products are available in various forms, including gels, creams, and suppositories, and can be applied directly to the vaginal area as needed.

Another option is hormone therapy, which involves using estrogen-based medications to restore vaginal moisture and elasticity. Estrogen therapy can be administered in the form of vaginal creams, tablets, or rings, and may provide relief from symptoms of vaginal dryness and discomfort. However, it's important to discuss the risks and benefits of hormone therapy with your healthcare provider, as it may not be suitable for everyone.

In addition to these treatments, practicing good vaginal hygiene and avoiding irritants such as perfumed soaps, douches, and harsh chemicals can help maintain vaginal health and reduce discomfort. Drinking plenty of water, staying sexually active, and using relaxation techniques to reduce stress can also support overall vaginal health and improve sexual satisfaction.

Strategies for Enhancing Intimacy and Pleasure

Communicate openly with your partner about your needs, desires, and concerns. Share your feelings and preferences openly, and encourage your partner to do the same. Effective communication can help build trust, intimacy, and mutual understanding in your relationship.

Explore new ways to experience pleasure and intimacy together, such as sensual massage, cuddling, or trying new sexual positions. Experimenting with different forms of touch and stimulation can help reignite passion and excitement in your relationship.

Prioritize self-care and relaxation to reduce stress and anxiety, which can interfere with sexual desire and arousal. Engage in activities that promote relaxation and pleasure, such as yoga, meditation, or spending quality time with your partner.

Invest in quality time together outside of the bedroom, such as going on romantic dates, taking walks in nature, or engaging in shared hobbies and interests. Building emotional connection and intimacy outside of sexual activity can strengthen your bond as a couple and enhance your overall relationship satisfaction.

Seek support from a therapist or counsellor if you're experiencing challenges in your relationship or struggling with sexual issues. Professional guidance can provide you with tools, strategies, and insights to navigate difficulties and improve your sexual health and satisfaction.

By implementing these strategies and exploring new ways to connect with your partner, you can enhance intimacy, pleasure, and satisfaction in your sexual relationship during menopause and beyond.

Chapter 8: Embracing Change and Finding Joy

Embracing the Journey of Menopause

Menopause is a journey, a new chapter in your life story. It's natural to feel uncertain or apprehensive about the changes happening in your body and your life. But remember, menopause is not an ending; it's a transition—a doorway to new possibilities. Embrace this journey with open arms. Take time to listen to your body and honour its needs. Embrace the wisdom that comes with experience and allow yourself to grow through this process.

You are embarking on a journey of self-discovery and transformation. Embrace it fully, knowing that you have the strength and resilience to navigate whatever challenges come your way.

Finding Joy and Purpose Beyond Menopause

Menopause marks the beginning of a new chapter—one filled with opportunities for growth, joy, and fulfilment. As you navigate this transition, take the time to reconnect with your passions, interests, and dreams.

Explore new hobbies, pursue creative endeavours, or reconnect with old friends. Find joy in the simple moments of life—whether it's enjoying a cup of tea, taking a walk in nature, or spending time with loved ones.

Remember that menopause is not the end of your journey; it's a new beginning. Find purpose in sharing your wisdom and experiences with others, and embrace the opportunity to live your life with intention and authenticity.

Celebrating Your Strength and Resilience

Menopause can be challenging, but it's also an opportunity to celebrate your strength and resilience. You've overcome obstacles and navigated through life's ups and downs, and now you're facing this new phase with courage and determination. Take pride in how far you've come and all that you've accomplished.

Celebrate the wisdom that comes with age and the resilience that has carried you through difficult times. Surround yourself with supportive friends and family who appreciate and admire your strength. And most importantly, celebrate yourself—your journey, your experiences, and the incredible woman you've become. You are strong, you are resilient, and you are worthy of celebration.

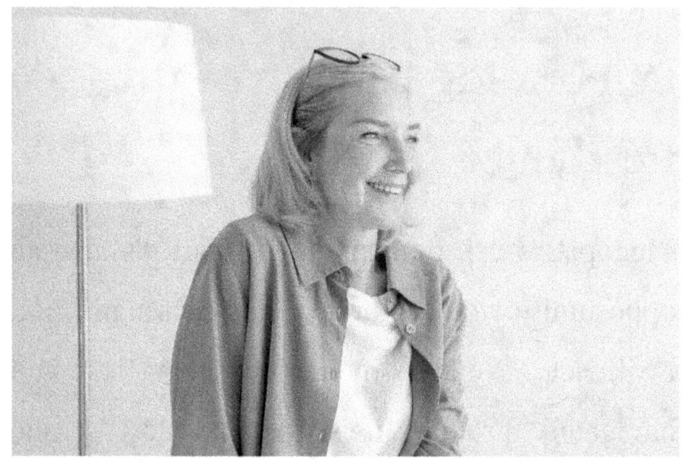

Conclusion

As you reflect on the wealth of knowledge and insights gained throughout this book, it's important to recognize the profound strength and resilience within you.

Menopause is not merely a passage marked by physical changes and hormonal fluctuations; it is a testament to the remarkable resilience of the female body and spirit. It's a time of transition, growth, and self-discovery—a journey that invites you to embrace change with an open heart and an unwavering sense of courage.

As you navigate the ups and downs of menopause, remember that you are not alone. Countless women around the world are experiencing the same challenges and triumphs, sharing in the collective wisdom and support of a sisterhood bound by shared experiences. Lean on your community, seek solace in the stories of others, and know that you are part of a tribe of women who understand and empathise with your journey.

Embrace the changes that come your way with grace and acceptance, recognizing that each shift, challenge, and triumph is an integral part of your evolution as a woman. Embrace your unique journey, celebrating the wisdom and insight that comes with age and experience.

As you close the pages of this book, may you carry with you the knowledge that you are capable, you are resilient, and you are never alone. Embrace the change, embrace your journey, and embrace the extraordinary woman that you are. The best is yet to come.

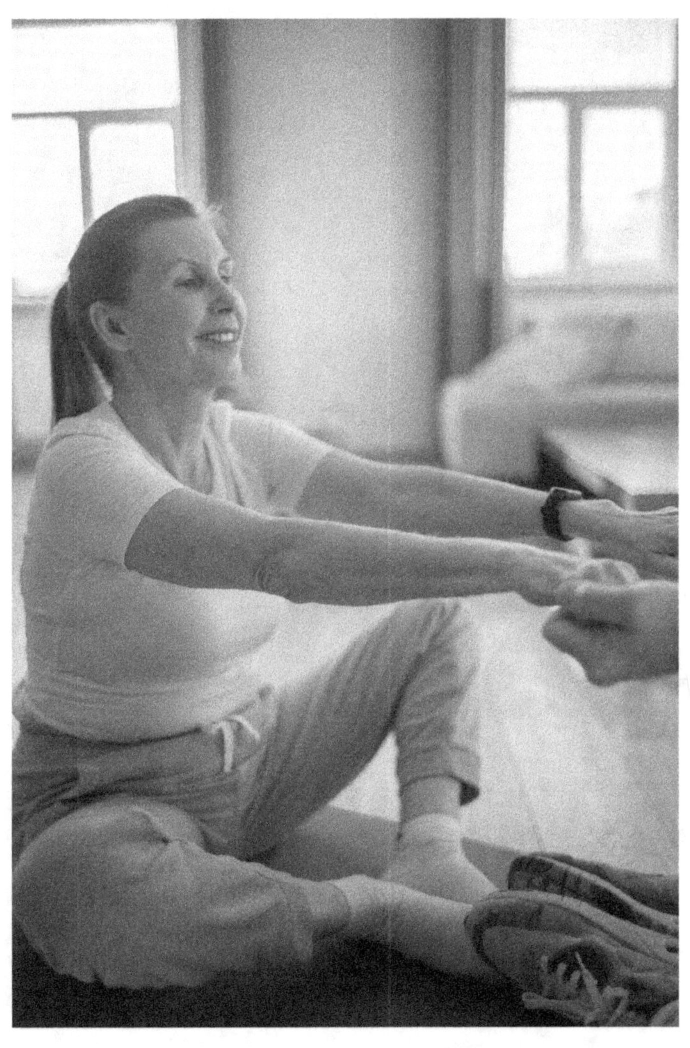